30 Day Intermittent Fasting Challenge:

Lose Weight and Accelerate Fat Loss with Intermittent Fasting

By
Nancy Wilson

Tale of Contents

Introduction: Are We Getting Fatter?

In modern society, it seems that no matter what we do, every single year—to be perfectly blunt—we are getting fatter. Societies of the industrial world continue to collectively gain more and more weight. Just to give you an idea of how much fatter, a research study conducted in 1975 revealed that approximately 105 million people could be considered morbidly obese worldwide, the same research was then repeated in 2014 and revealed that the globe obesity index for that year was 641 million!

And in the years since this 2014 study we can only assume that the number has risen even higher. Just look at China. No one ever imagined that this major bastion of the orient where for thousands of years lean eating was ingrained in the cultural consciousness, would one day face an obesity problem. But the numbers don't lie—China has in fact just surpassed the United States as the most obese country on the planet! Upon hearing such things, a few snap judgements could be made about China's eager importation of American fast food as the reason behind this.

But even though the golden arches of McDonalds and the spinning chicken buckets of KFC being established all up and down the Silk Road no doubt play a part—it can't all be blamed on fast food alone.

There is an overall eating lifestyle that has impacted how we eat, and even how we digest food. The issue at hand is not so much a matter of willing ourselves not to eat, and an inability to restrict calories—the real problem is erratic eating habits within a chaotic lifestyle. In order to be successful at any diet, you need to commit yourself to a meal plan that will work for you and your schedule.

The reason why fad diets don't work is precisely that—they are fads! They are designed to help you lose a few pounds after a few weeks, but they are unsustainable for the long haul. The only way we can really lose weight and keep that fat at bay is by following sustainable models of diet and wellness that we can follow for the rest of our lives. The intermittent fast diet provides you with just that. Follow along with us in this book as we take you through a 30 Day Intermittent Fasting Challenge, and on down a path of long lived health and wellness.

Chapter 1: It's All About Insulin

Insulin, a hormone created by the pancreas, is nothing short of a naturally produced wonder-drug. The body depends on the production of insulin in order to help store up energy, regulate blood sugar, and to facilitate human growth. Indeed, a lack, or shortage of insulin is what leads to the debilitating illness of diabetes. But overproduction of insulin can be just as problematic, since it is insulin that regulates fat storage. High levels of insulin send a signal to the body to begin storing fat deposits as energy. It's a fairly simple calculus; the more insulin—the more fat!

You see as our insulin levels rise, so does levels of fat within our cells. Under lower insulin conditions, fat is able to squeeze through cell walls and disperse on out of the body as waste. But as insulin begins to be stockpiled in the body, fat storage is encouraged, causing the very walls of our cells to stiffen and not allow that fat to leave. These numerous cells hanging on to your fat for dear life are what eventually manifest as cellulite, muffin tops, and all manner of other stubborn body fat that you just can't seem to get rid of.

Since insulin is such a controller of these bodily functions, then doesn't it make sense to try and control insulin? This is precisely what sets the intermittent fasting diet apart from others. This diet serves as a concerted effort to reprogram the body, learning to manipulate our very levels of insulin so that we can keep the body from storing so much fat. This form of dieting takes a look at the source of the malady rather than simply treating the symptoms.

We get to the root cause, and work to eliminate it. You see, the absence of food during fasting automatically lowers our insulin, encouraging our cells to soften up and let fat out so that we can burn it up as energy. This is a good thing, but excessive fasting for several days at a time, will ultimately backfire on us, because although it lowers insulin it will alter the course of our metabolism. This is why an intermittent fast of fasting one day, and then eating normally the next has been proven to be ideal. This will help keep both your insulin and your metabolism in check.

Chapter 2: Choose Your "Eating Window"

The most important thing to grasp when it comes to an intermittent fast is the fact that there are specific "eating windows" to which the dieter should adhere in order to maximize their success with their meal plans. What are these eating windows? Strictly speaking—an eating window is simply referring to the "time when you can consume food" when you are *not fasting*. You see whenever it is that you are actively eating, it is said that you are within a "fed state".

During this period your bodily metabolic processes are running full steam ahead, making short work of the food you eat, utilizing nutrients, storing fat, and streamlining waste. But it is when your body is in its "fasting state" that the fat stores really begin to burn. But for the purpose of this book we will refer to the active eating state as your eating window. For some who fast, their fasting window may only last the first 12 hours of their day with a light meal of 500 calories or less in the evening.

But others may indeed go for the whole 24 hours, not eating anything at all during that particular fasting window. If you are going to do a 12 hour fast, this means that the eating window is 12 hours as well. But if you go for the full 24-hour fast, then the next corresponding day you will have a matching eating window expanded to 24 hours here too. As you can see, it all balances out either way you do it. It's just a matter of what works best for you. Some find it easier to fast completely one day and eat the next. Many find it easier to not have to calorie count at the end of the day for a meal under 500 calories.

For them it is simply a cut and dry affair of *Monday I eat*, then *Tuesday I don't*. But if you would rather pace yourself with a 12-hour intermittent fast, that means you will have to be more careful with your following 12-hour window, making sure to prepare healthy and fresh meals of less than 500 calories for the remainder of your evening. However, you wish to do it, the eating window needs to match up with your fasting window. These are just a few brief examples however, and there are many more eating windows to choose from. Here they are a little bit more in depth.

Crescendo Method

This method is great for those that wish to get themselves used to the fasting regimen on an incremental basis. Rather than jumping in all at once, the Crescendo Method allows you to simply wade in the water. This can be beneficial if you have a rather sensitive system, and worry about creating an imbalance in hormones and metabolic function. This method spaces out fasting throughout the week in a stacked fashion that is truly intermittent, such as fasting Tuesday, Thursday, and Saturday, and eating on the days in between.

16/8 Method

This fasting method has been created to specifically target fat in the body. It helps you to improve muscle mass, as well as burn up fat! What you do is you set aside a window of time within which to fast for about 16 hours, and then you establish a following window of time in which you can eat consisting of the next 8 hours. Just to be clear, you aren't supposed to overindulge and pig out for 8 hours straight! The 8-hour window is simply the approximate amount of time in which you can plan, cook, and eat your healthy low-fat meals.

24 Hour Protocol

This fasting method has been popular for a while now and requires the dieter to basically "eat stop eat" a few times a week. It's up to you what time you fast, and what time you begin to eat again. Just follow the 24-hour protocol and you will be doing just fine in no time! This is actually my preferred method for the intermittent fast, I find that I can easily go a whole day without eating when I know I have the whole next day to recuperate.

5:2 Diet

You may have heard of this fasting method before. As the name just might imply, this fasting method involves the restriction of calories for 2 days out of the week, and then eating normally for the other 5. Many enjoy the makeup of this regimen, since it enables them to do things such as eat what they want on the weekend, while fasting on Monday and Tuesday. Conversely, others like to fast through Saturday and Sunday, while eating normally during the rest of their week. In the end it is up to you to choose the exact intermittent fasting strategy that works best for you and your schedule.

Chapter 3: Breakfast for Your Intermittent Fast

Breakfast is the most important meal of the day, and the same can still very much be said during your intermittent fasting routine. Breakfast is what gets us up and going in the morning, so don't deprive yourself! Here in this chapter we will provide you with just the meals you need to keep you healthy and satisfied throughout the course of your day!

Green Eggs and Bacon

Who needs green eggs and ham when you can have Green Eggs and Bacon? This recipe comes fully loaded with eggs and bacon, as well as avocado, almonds, garlic, and a clever mixture of spice to make everything all nice.

Prep Time: 5 min

Passive Time: 0 min

Cook Time: 5 min

Total: 10 min

Serves: 3-4

Ingredients:
- 2 eggs
- 3 slices of bacon
- 1 tablespoon of olive oil
- 1 avocado
- 1 tsp of salt
- 1 tsp of pepper
- 1 tablespoon of pesto
- ¼ cup of almonds
- 1 tablespoon of chopped basil
- 1 tablespoon of olive oil

- 2 tablespoons of lemon juice
- 1 tablespoon of chopped garlic
- 1 tsp of coconut oil

Directions:

1. Get out a medium sized frying pan and add your 2 eggs, your 3 slices of bacon, and your tablespoon of olive oil.

2. Set your burner to medium heat, and stir the ingredients into the oil as they cook for about 2 minutes.

3. Now add your tsp of salt, your tsp of pepper, your tablespoon of pesto, and your ¼ cup of almonds to the pan.

4. Stir and cook for another 5 minutes.

5. Now place your avocado onto a clean cutting board, and quarter them into slices.

6. Place on a plate, add your bacon and eggs, and serve!

Morning Casserole

Wake up in the morning to this fantastic casserole! With eggs, spaghetti squash, heavy cream, and cheddar cheese, this dish comes packed with tremendous flavor!

Prep Time: 5 min

Passive Time: 0 min

Cook Time: 25 min

Total: 30 min

Serves: 5-6

Ingredients:
- 2 cups of cooked spaghetti squash
- 12 eggs
- 1 cup of heavy cream
- 1 cup of shredded cheddar cheese

Directions:
1. Go ahead and set your oven for 375 degrees.
2. While your oven is heating up, take out a mixing bowl and add your 2 cups of cooked spaghetti squash, your 12 eggs, your cup of heavy cream, and your cup of shredded cheddar cheese.

3. Stir these ingredients together well, and pour them into a casserole dish.
4. Place the dish into your oven and allow the ingredients to cook for about 25 minutes.
5. Serve when ready.

Egg, Veggie, and Beef Frittata

So, you say want to eat right and lose the fat? Well—with just the right kick of eggs, vegetables, and beef, this Frittata has breakfast down pat!

Prep Time: 2 min

Passive Time: 0 min

Cook Time: 8 min

Total: 10 min

Serves: 2

Ingredients:
- 2 tsp of coconut oil
- ¼ cup of chopped onion
- ½ pound of ground beef
- ½ cup of crumbled, cooked bacon
- ½ cup of chopped tomatoes
- 1 cup of chopped spinach
- ½ tsp of salt
- 1 tsp of pepper
- 3 eggs

Directions:
1. First, set your oven to 355 degrees.

2. While your oven is heating get out two sheets of aluminum foil.

3. Place a large frying pan onto a burner set for high heat and add your 2 tsp of coconut oil, your ¼ cup of chopped onion, and your ½ pound of ground beef.

4. Stir and cook these ingredients for about 5 minutes

5. Next, add in your cup of chopped tomatoes, your cup of chopped spinach, and season on top with your ½ tsp of salt, and tsp of pepper.

6. Stir and cook for another 3 minutes.

7. After this, get out a medium sized mixing bowl and add your 3 eggs, stirring them together.

8. Pour your cooked meat mixture into the medium sized mixing bowl, and stir all of the ingredients together.

9. Deposit this combined mixture back into your frying pan, and cook for about 10 minutes on each side.

10. Serve when ready.

Eggs in Limbo

If you need a good and satisfying breakfast in the morning, this dish has it. Loaded with onions, garlic, tomatoes, and eggs, you've got everything you need to start your day. So don't just stare at your plate with your elbows all akimbo, put a fork and knife in those hands, and dig into this netherworld of breakfast— Eggs in Limbo!

Prep Time: 4 min

Passive Time: 0 min

Cook Time: 8 min

Total: 12 min

Serves: 1-2

Ingredients:
- 1 tablespoon of olive oil
- ½ cup of chopped onions
- 1 tsp of chopped garlic
- 1 cup of chopped tomatoes
- 1 tsp of pepper
- 3 tablespoons of chopped basil
- 4 eggs

Directions:

1. Place a medium sized frying pan onto a burner set for medium heat and add your tablespoon of olive oil, followed by your ½ cup of chopped onions, your tsp of chopped garlic, your cup of chopped tomatoes and your tsp of ground pepper.

2. Stir and cook these ingredients over the course of the next 5 minutes.

3. Next, add your 4 eggs, and stir them into the mix, cooking another 3 minutes.

4. Finally, turn off the burner, top with your 3 tablespoons of chopped basil.

5. Your Eggs in Limbo are ready!

Cheddar Biscuits

Settle in for some Cheddar Biscuits and Gravy! With a healthy helping of eggs, garlic, almond flour, and sea salt, this dish has just what your craving! A little bit of cheddar makes everything better!

Prep Time: 5 min

Passive Time: 0 min

Cook Time: 12 min

Total: 17 min

Serves: 2-3

Ingredients:
- 3 eggs
- 1 tablespoon of chopped garlic
- 1 cup of almond flour
- 1 tsp of baking powder
- ½ tsp of sea salt
- 2 tablespoons of unsalted butter
- ½ cup of sharp cheddar cheese

Directions:
1. Set your oven for 420 degrees.
2. While the oven heats up, get out a medium sized mixing bowl and add your 3 eggs,

followed by your tablespoon of chopped garlic, stir together and place to the side.

3. Now get out another bowl and add your cup of almond flour, your tsp of baking powder, and your ½ tsp of sea salt, stirring everything together well.

4. Next, add your 2 tablespoons of unsalted butter, and your ½ cup of sharp cheddar cheese.

5. Use your (clean) hands to shape your biscuits. You should be able to make eight.

6. Place your eight biscuits onto the cooking sheet and put them into the oven.

7. Bake for about 12 minutes.

8. Serve immediately.

Almond and Coconut Flour Pancakes

You won't be late for breakfast with this recipe on the menu! You are going to love the taste of these great pancakes!

Prep Time: 4 min

Passive Time: 0 min

Cook Time: 4 min

Total: 8 min

Serves: 2-3

Ingredients:
- ½ cup of coconut flour
- 2 cups of almond flour
- 1 tablespoon of sugar
- ½ tsp of baking powder
- ½ tsp of sea salt
- 1 cup of almond milk
- 2 tablespoons of melted butter
- 1 tsp of vanilla extract
- 7 large eggs

Directions:

1. Get out a large mixing bowl and add your ½ cup of coconut flour, your 2 cups of almond flour, your tablespoon of sugar, your ½ tsp of baking powder, and your ½ tsp of sea salt.

2. Now get out another bowl and add your 2 cups of almond milk, your 2 tablespoons of melted butter, your tsp of vanilla extract, and your 7 eggs.

3. Stir this bowl of ingredients together before adding it to the other bowl of ingredients.

4. Stir everything together, this completes your pancake batter.

5. Put about one clump of batter for each pancake you make.

6. Place your pancake clumps into a large frying pan, and cook 2 minutes on each side under high heat.

7. Serve when ready.

Granola and Cinnamon

Are you tired of complex recipes that take too much of your time? Well then, if that's the case—for a simple and easy breakfast, that takes just the bare minimum, try this tasty batch of Granola and Cinnamon! You will be glad you did!

Prep Time: 5 min and 45 seconds

Passive Time: 0 min

Cook Time: 20 min

Total: 25 min and 45 seconds

Serves: 3-4

Ingredients:
- 2 tablespoons of chia seeds
- 3 tablespoons of water
- ½ tsp of vanilla extract
- ½ cup of macadamia nuts
- 1 tablespoon of whey protein powder
- 2 tablespoons of flaxseed meal
- 1 tsp of cinnamon
- ½ tsp of salt
- 2 tablespoons of melted coconut oil

Directions:

1. Set your oven's temperature to 355 degrees.

2. Now get out a medium sized mixing bowl and add your 2 tablespoons of chia seeds, your 3 tablespoons of water, and your ½ tsp of vanilla extract and stir them all together well.

3. Next, take your ½ cup of macadamia nuts, your tablespoon of whey protein powder, your 2 tablespoons of flaxseed meal, your tsp of cinnamon, and your ½ tsp of salt, and add them to a blender.

4. Blend for about 45 seconds.

5. Deposit the mixture onto a piece of parchment, on a cooking sheet, and use your (clean) hands to flatten it.

6. Place into the oven and cook for 15 minutes

7. Take out of the oven and layer the contents of your other mixing bowl—the chia mixture over the ingredients already on the sheet.

8. Place back into the oven and cook for another 5 minutes.

9. After your 5 minutes have passed, take the sheet out of the oven, cut into squares, and serve.

Bowl of Morning Porridge

As we struggle to get up and moving in the morning, many of us are reaching for the coffee pot to get a dose of our *morning courage*. But besides coffee, this Bowl of Morning Porridge, is also good to give you the boost you need to go about your day with confidence!

Prep Time: 5 min

Passive Time: 0 min

Cook Time: 20 min

Total: 25 min

Serves: 2-3

Ingredients:
- 4 tablespoons of shredded coconut
- 1 tablespoon of oat bran
- 1 tablespoon of flaxseed meal
- ½ tablespoon of butter
- 1 tablespoon of sugar
- 1 tsp of cinnamon
- ½ cup of heavy cream
- 1 cup of water
- 1 tsp of salt

Directions:

1. Place a small pot on a burner set to high heat, and add your 4 tablespoons of shredded coconut, followed by your tablespoon of oat bran, your tablespoon of flaxseed meal, your ½ tablespoon of butter, your tablespoon of sugar, your tsp of cinnamon, your ½ cup of heavy cream, your cup of water, and your tsp of salt.

2. Stir and mix the entire contents of the pot, as it cooks over the course of the next 20 minutes.

3. Serve when ready.

Chapter 4: A Bit of Lunch Cuisine In Between

When the lunch hour strikes, don't wreck your *fast* by reaching for *fast food*! Don't let those burgers and fries go to your head (or your stomach), Try some of these healthy alternatives instead! You're going to love it!

Beefy Green Lettuce Wraps

Beef and all the fixings wrapped up in a piece of lettuce! This dish is so good, don't be surprised if you want to dive right in. Go ahead and pack this mean bit of green for your lunch my friend!

Prep Time: 3 min

Passive Time: 0 min

Cook Time: 7 min

Total: 10 min

Serves: 3-4

Ingredients:
- 1 tablespoon of olive oil
- 2 tablespoons of chopped onions
- ½ tsp of chopped garlic
- 1 tsp of chili powder
- 1-pound lean ground beef
- 1 tablespoon of chopped cilantro
- 1 tablespoon of chopped parsley
- ½ tsp of sea salt
- 1 tsp of pepper
- ½ cup of chopped tomatoes

- ½ cup of chopped cucumbers
- 1 tablespoon of lemon juice
- ½ tsp of cayenne pepper
- ½ tsp of sea salt
- 1 cup of chopped avocado
- 4 Romaine lettuce leaves

Directions:

1. In a medium sized frying pan add your tablespoon of olive oil, evenly distributing it, and set the burner for medium heat.

2. Next, add in your 2 tablespoons of chopped onions, your ½ tsp of chopped garlic, your tsp of chili powder, and stir and cook for about 2 minutes.

3. After this, add in your pound of lean ground beef, stir and cook for another 5 minutes.

4. While cooking, get out a medium sized mixing bowl and add your tablespoon of chopped parsley, your ½ tsp of sea salt your tsp of pepper, your ½ cup of chopped tomatoes, your ½ cup of chopped cucumbers, your tablespoon of lemon juice, your ½ tsp of cayenne pepper, your ½ tsp of sea salt, your cup of chopped avocado. Mix together well.

5. Now go back to your meat mixture and scoop it up into your romaine leaves.

6. Finally, add your mixing bowl topping on top of the meat, wrap the lettuce leaves up tight, and your Beefy Green Lettuce Wraps are ready!

Mushroom, Chicken, and Veggie Stir Fry

If you are looking for a good lunch, I have a suggestion—Mushroom, chicken and all of your favorite vegetables stir fried to perfection!

Prep Time: 2 min

Passive Time: 0 min

Cook Time: 8 min

Total: 10 min

Serves: 2

Ingredients:
- 2 tsp of coconut oil
- 1 tsp of chopped ginger
- ½ tsp of chopped garlic
- ½ tsp of red pepper
- 1 cup of chopped chicken
- ½ cup of chopped mushrooms
- 1 cup of shredded cabbage
- ½ cup of chopped carrots
- ½ cup of chopped celery
- ½ cup of chopped green bell pepper
- 1 tablespoon of coconut oil

- 1 tsp of sea salt
- 1 tsp of pepper
- 1 tsp of sesame seeds

Directions:

1. In a medium sized frying pan add your 2 tsp of coconut oil, and set the burner for high heat.

2. Now add your tsp of chopped ginger, your ½ tsp of chopped garlic, your ½ tsp of red pepper, and your cup of chopped chicken.

3. Stir and cook these ingredients for about 4 minutes, before adding in your ½ cup of chopped mushrooms, and cooking for 1 more minute.

4. Next, add your cup of shredded cabbage, followed by your ½ cup of celery, your ½ cup of chopped green bell pepper, your tablespoon of coconut oil, your tsp of sea salt, your tsp of pepper, and your tsp of sesame seeds.

5. Stir everything together and cook over the course of the next 3 minutes.

6. Serve when ready.

Turkey Lettuce Burgers

You can take the wholesome taste of meatloaf and roll it up into these delicious Turkey Lettuce Burgers! If you are hungry and need something that will fill you up right, give this recipe a try!

Prep Time: 5 min

Passive Time: 0 min

Cook Time: 5 min

Total: 10 min

Serves: 2

Ingredients:
- 1 pound of ground turkey
- 2 egg whites
- ¼ cup of chopped onion
- 3 tablespoons of tomato sauce
- 1 tablespoon of chopped garlic
- ¼ tsp of dried oregano
- ½ tsp of salt
- 2 slices of tomato
- 4 large leaves of lettuce
- 2 tablespoons of Dijon Mustard

Directions:

1. In a medium sized mixing bowl add your pound of ground turkey, your 2 egg whites, your ¼ cup of chopped onion, your 3 tablespoons of chopped garlic, your ¼ tsp of dried oregano, and your ½ tsp of salt.

2. Now take your (clean) hands and use them to press the ingredients into 2 separate patties.

3. Place a medium sized frying pan onto a burner set for high heat and deposit your 2 patties onto the pan.

4. Cook for about 5 minutes on each side.

5. While cooking lay out your lettuce leaves on two separate plates.

6. Place the cooked burger on one of the leaves, and top each one with 1 slice of lettuce and 1 tablespoon of Dijon Mustard.

7. Now place the remaining leaf on each hamburger.

8. Your Turkey Lettuce Burgers are ready to eat!

Cod and Olives

This recipe will have you back for seconds! Have a light lunch of fish, olives, and tomato!

Prep Time: 5 min

Passive Time: 0 min

Cook Time: 15 min

Total: 20 min

Serves: 1-2

Ingredients:
- 1 tablespoon of olive oil
- ½ cup of chopped onion
- 1 tsp of chopped garlic
- ½ cup of chopped green bell pepper
- 1 tsp of dried oregano
- 2 tablespoons of chopped green olives
- ½ tsp of ground cinnamon
- 1 cup of chopped tomatoes
- 1 tablespoon of chopped parsley
- ½ cup of water
- ½ tsp of salt
- 1 tsp of pepper
- ½ pound of fresh cod

Directions:

1. Inside a large frying pan add your tablespoon of olive oil, your ½ cup of chopped onion, your tsp of chopped garlic, and your ½ cup of chopped green bell pepper.

2. Stir and cook these ingredients together for about 5 minutes.

3. Next, add your tsp of dried oregano, your 2 tablespoons of chopped green olives, and your ½ tsp of ground cinnamon, followed by your cup of chopped tomatoes, tablespoon of chopped parsley, and your ½ cup of water.

4. Stir and cook for another 5 minutes.

5. After this add your ½ tsp of salt, your tsp of pepper, and your ½ pound of fresh cod.

6. Stir and cook these ingredients together for another 5 minutes.

7. Turn your burner off, and serve.

Lettuce Lamb Tacos

This meal may not be all that macho. But whether you are taking a lunch break or simply out on the lamb with some friends, you are going to love these Lettuce Lamb Tacos.

Prep Time: 7 min

Passive Time: 0 min

Cook Time: 5 min

Total: 12 min

Serves: 2-4

Ingredients:
- 1 tablespoon of olive oil
- 2 tablespoons of chopped onion
- ¼ tsp of chopped garlic
- 1 pound of ground lamb
- 1 tablespoon of fresh mint
- 1 tablespoon of parsley
- ½ tsp of sea salt
- ¼ tsp of fresh ground pepper
- 4 Romaine lettuce leaves
- 1 cup of chopped tomato
- 1 cup of chopped cucumber

- 1 lemon wedge

Directions:

1. Place a large frying pan on a burner set for high heat.

2. Now add your 2 tablespoons of chopped onion, and your ¼ tsp of chopped garlic, and stir and cook the ingredients for 2 minutes.

3. Next add your pound of ground lamb, followed by your tablespoon of fresh mint, your tablespoon of parsley, your ½ tsp of sea salt, your ¼ tsp of fresh ground pepper, and cook for 3 more minutes.

4. Now lay out your 4 lettuce leaves onto plates, and add your meat mixture to each lettuce leaf.

5. Top off the meat by evenly distributing your cup of chopped tomato, and your cup of chopped cucumber.

6. Finally, squeeze your lemon wedge over each, fold the lettuce over like a taco, and serve.

Chicken Stir Fry

You know what they say—little bit of stir fry can really go a long way! And with this delicious dish, this is most certainly the case!

Prep Time: 2 min

Passive Time: 0 min

Cook Time: 8 min

Total: 10 min

Serves: 2-3

Ingredients:
- 2 cups of shredded chicken
- 1 tablespoon of soy sauce
- 2 tablespoons of olive oil
- 1 tsp of grated ginger
- ½ cup of diced green bell pepper
- 1 cup of rice, cooked

Directions:
1. Place a medium sized frying pan on a burner set for medium-high heat, and add your 2 tablespoons of olive oil to the pan.

2. Now add your 2 cups of shredded chicken followed by your tablespoon of soy sauce, and your tsp of grated ginger.

3. Stir and cook the ingredients for about 5 minutes, before adding your ½ cup of diced green bell pepper, and cup of cooked rice.

4. Stir and cook all the ingredients together for about 3 more minutes.

5. Serve when ready.

Fire Chicken

Chicken breasts, tabasco, and sour cream—put some fire in your lunchtime routine!

Prep Time: 5 min

Passive Time: 0 min

Cook Time: 45 min

Total: 50 min

Serves: 1-2

Ingredients:
- 2 chicken breasts
- 1 cup of sour cream
- 2 tsp of tabasco sauce
- ½ tsp of celery salt
- ½ tsp of black pepper

Directions:
1. Set your oven for 355 degrees, grease a cooking sheet and set it to the side.
2. Now get out a small mixing bowl and add your cup of sour cream, your 2 tsp of tabasco sauce, your ½ tsp of celery salt, and your ½ tsp of black pepper.
3. Stir the ingredients together well.

4. Lay out your 2 chicken breasts on the cooking sheet and pour the sour cream mixture over the chicken breasts.

5. Put the cooking sheet in the oven and cook for about 45 minutes.

6. Once cooked, take out of the oven immediately, and serve.

Chapter 5: Dinner Meals After the Fast

If you have ever went to sleep hungry, you know just how hard those nighttime hunger pains can be. It is for this reason that how we end our day during a fast is just as important as how we begin it. Here in this chapter you will find a listing of healthy but hearty meals with which you can partake for your evening diner meal after you finish up your fasting.

Cheesy Meatloaf Dinner

Meatloaf is a mainstay, comfort food classic, and you will find this Cheesy Meatloaf Dinner to be absolutely fantastic!

Prep Time: 5 min

Passive Time: 0 min

Cook Time: 25 min

Total: 30 min

Serves: 1-2

Ingredients:
- 1 pound of ground beef
- ¼ cup of chopped onion
- 1 tablespoon of chopped garlic
- 1 cup of flaxmeal
- 2 tablespoons of coconut oil
- 4 tablespoons of unsweetened tomato passata
- 1 tablespoon of dried herbs
- ¼ cup of chopped green pepper
- ½ cup of shredded cheddar cheese
- ¼ cup of shredded Gouda cheese
- ½ cup of parmesan cheese

Directions:

1. Set your oven for 355 degrees.

2. While your oven is heating up, deposit your pound of ground beef, your ¼ cup of chopped onion, your tablespoon of chopped garlic, and your cup of flaxmeal into a large bowl and stir together.

3. Now add your 2 tablespoons of coconut oil, your 4 tablespoons of unsweetened tomato passata, and your tablespoon of dried herbs and stir everything together well.

4. Get out a greased cooking sheet and spread your ingredients over the bottom of it.

5. Follow this up by laying out your ½ cup of shredded cheddar cheese, and ¼ cup of shredded Gouda cheese over the meat spread.

6. Now sprinkle your ½ cup of parmesan cheese on top.

7. Place in the oven and cook for about 25 minutes.

1. Slice and serve.

Salty Beef Tenderloin and Mushrooms

Eating this dish after a fast won't tie your stomach into knots, this salty beef really hits the spot!

Prep Time: 11 min

Passive Time: 0 min

Cook Time: 9 min

Total: 20 min

Serves: 2

Ingredients:
- 4 cups of chopped cauliflower
- ¼ cup of water
- ½ pound of beef tenderloin
- 1 cup of chopped mushrooms
- ½ tsp of salt
- 1 tsp of fresh thyme
- ¼ tsp of ground pepper

Directions:
1. In a heat resistant bowl place your 4 cups of chopped cauliflower, and your ¼ cup of water.

46

2. Wrap the bowl in plastic wrap and place in the microwave, cooking the ingredients for 4 minutes.

3. Now place a large frying pan onto a burner set for high heat and put your ½ pound of beef tenderloin into the pan.

4. Next, add your cup of chopped mushrooms, and cook the meat for about 5 minutes on each side.

5. Season with a ½ tsp of fresh thyme, and a ½ tsp of salt.

6. Dish up your meat and mushrooms on a plate and serve with a side of cauliflower.

Pork Chop Feast

Pork chops provide a filling feast after your fast!

Prep Time: 5 min

Passive Time: 0 min

Cook Time: 45 min

Total: 50 min

Serves: 2-3

Ingredients:
- 7 pork chops
- ½ cup of diced onion
- ¼ cup of diced tomato
- 1 tsp of pepper
- 1 tsp of salt
- 1 tablespoon of olive oil

Directions:
1. Preheat your oven to 390 degrees.
2. Get out a large cooking sheet and grease it with your tablespoon of olive oil.
3. Spread out your 7 pork chops over the cooking sheet.

4. Now add your ½ cup of diced onion, and your ¼ cup of diced tomato to the cooking sheet.

5. Season with your tsp of salt, and tsp of pepper, and put cooking sheet into the oven.

6. Cook for 45 minutes.

7. Once cooked, serve immediately.

Taco Casserole

You'll want to eat it as soon as you take it out of the oven!

Prep Time: 5 min

Passive Time: 0 min

Cook Time: 45 min

Total: 50 min

Serves: 3-4

Ingredients:
- 1 pound of ground turkey
- ¼ cup of chopped cauliflower
- ¼ cup of chopped jalapeno
- ¼ cup of chopped red bell peppers
- ¼ cup of chopped onion
- 1 tsp of cumin
- 1 tsp of parsley
- 1 tsp of turmeric
- 1 tsp of chopped garlic
- 1 tsp of oregano
- 1 cup of shredded cheddar cheese

Directions:

1. Take out a large mixing bowl and add your pound of ground turkey, followed by your 1 tsp of cumin, your 1 tsp of parsley, your 1 tsp of turmeric, your 1 tsp of chopped garlic, and your 1 tsp of oregano, and stir together well.

2. Next, add your ¼ cup of chopped cauliflower, your ¼ cup of chopped jalapeno, your ¼ cup of chopped red bell peppers, and your ¼ cup of chopped onion.

3. Briefly stir all of the ingredients before pouring them into a casserole dish.

4. Sprinkle your cup of shredded cheddar cheese on top of the ingredients in the dish.

5. Place in the oven, set the temperature for 400 degrees, and cook for 45 minutes.

6. Serve immediately!

Portobello Philly Cheesesteak

It's Philly Cheesesteak stuffed inside a Portobello mushroom!

Prep Time: 5 min

Passive Time: 0 min

Cook Time: 7 min

Total: 12 min

Serves: 4

Ingredients:
- 6 ounces of sliced sirloin steaks
- ½ tsp of kosher salt
- 1 tsp of black pepper
- 1 cup of diced onion
- 1 cup of chopped green bell pepper
- 1 tablespoon of sour cream
- 2 tablespoons of mayonnaise
- 2 ounces of cream cheese
- 3 ounces of shredded provolone cheese
- 4 large Portobello mushrooms

Directions:
1. Set the temperature of your oven to 400 degrees.

2. While your oven is warming up take out your 4 large Portobello mushrooms, take out the stems, remove the gills, and season the caps with your ½ tsp of kosher salt, and your tsp of black pepper.

3. Put these to the side for a moment, and take a large frying pan and place it on a burner set for high heat.

4. Deposit your 6 ounces of sliced sirloin steaks into the pan, and cook for about 2 minutes on each side.

5. After this, add in your cup of diced onion, and your cup of chopped green bell pepper.

6. Stir and cook these ingredients together for another 3 minutes.

7. Next, place your Portobello mushroom caps on a greased cooking sheet and then spoon your cooked ingredients evenly into all 4 of the caps.

8. Place these stuffed caps into the oven and cook for about 400 degrees.

Beef Stew Supper

There is just something about Beef Stew after a long day of work! No matter what's going on around you, it feels you up and makes you feel alright!

Prep Time: 10 min

Passive Time: 0 min

Cook Time: 15 min

Total: 25 min

Serves: 3-4

Ingredients:
- 1 cup of chopped celery
- 1 cup of chopped carrots
- ½ cup of diced potatoes
- 2 cups of chopped onions
- 1 cup of tomato sauce
- 3 tablespoons of almond flour
- 1 tsp of salt
- 1 tsp of pepper
- 2 cups of beef broth
- 2 cups of shredded beef

Directions:

1. Place a large pot onto a burner set for medium-high heat and add your 2 cups of beef broth to the pan.

2. Let your broth heat up for 1 minute before adding your cup of chopped celery, your cup of chopped carrots, your ½ cup of diced potatoes, your 2 cups of chopped onions, and cup of tomato sauce.

3. Mix the ingredients together well for about 10 minutes before adding your 2 cups of shredded beef to the pot.

4. Stir in your 3 tablespoons of almond flour, then add your tsp of salt, and your tsp of pepper.

5. Continue to periodically stir the ingredients together over the course of the next 15 minutes.

6. After your 15 minutes have passed, serve whenever you are ready to do so.

Cheesy Chick Peas and Chicken Au Gratin

Scrumptious Chick Peas lend themselves to the classic flavorings of Chicken Au Gratin!

Prep Time: 2 min

Passive Time: 0 min

Cook Time: 4 min

Total: 6 min

Serves: 3-4

Ingredients:

- 1 cup of chick peas
- 1 cup of shredded chicken
- 1 can of cream of chicken
- ½ cup of water
- 1 tsp of salt
- 1 tsp of pepper
- 1 cup of shredded cheddar cheese

Directions:

1. Add your cup of chick peas, and your cup of shredded chicken to a medium sized sauce pan followed by the can of cream of chicken, your ½ cup of water, and your tsp of salt.

2. Now set your burner for high heat and stir the ingredients as they cook over the course of the next 4 minutes.

3. After your 4 minutes have passed, add in your cup of shredded cheddar cheese, stirring the cheese into the other ingredients over the next 2 minutes.

4. Finally, turn the burner off, season with your tsp of pepper, and serve.

Pizza Hot Pocket

Everybody likes pizza! Enough said!

Prep Time: 5 min

Passive Time: 0 min

Cook Time: 15 min

Total: 20 min

Serves: 1-2

Ingredients:

- 1 cup of shredded mozzarella cheese
- ½ cup of almond meal flour
- 2 tablespoons of cream cheese
- ½ tsp of salt
- 1 egg
- 2 tablespoons of tomato paste
- ½ cup of chopped mushrooms
- ¼ cup of diced green bell pepper

Directions:

1. In a medium sized mixing bowl add your cup of shredded mozzarella cheese, followed by your ½ cup of almond meal flour, and your 2 tablespoons of cream cheese.

2. Place the bowl into the microwave and cook the ingredients for about 45 seconds.

3. Take out the microwaved ingredients and add your egg, and ½ tsp of salt to the mix, stirring them together.

4. Now take your (clean) hands and knead the mixture into what will constitute your dough.

5. Now deposit your 2 tablespoons of tomato paste, your ½ cup of chopped mushrooms, and your ¼ cup of diced green bell pepper into the center of the dough, fold the dough over, and place it onto a greased cooking sheet and stick it into the oven.

6. Set your oven temperature for 400 degrees, and cook for 15 minutes.

7. Serve up this Pizza Hot Pocket while still hot!

Chapter 6: Soups, Snacks, Sides, and Salads for Fasting

As much as we would like to focus on what we are eating for our main course meals, sometimes it's the smaller entrees and additions that make all the difference. Here in this chapter you will find all of the best soups, sides, and salads to consume during your 30-Day Intermittent Fast Challenge.

Homemade Cream of Mushroom Soup

Just like mom used to make! Homemade Cream of Mushroom Soup!

Prep Time: 3 min

Passive Time: 0 min

Cook Time: 20 min

Total: 23 min

Serves: 1-2

Ingredients:
- 1 tablespoon of coconut oil
- 1 cup of chopped onions
- 1 tsp of chopped garlic
- ½ cup of chopped mushrooms
- 1 tsp of fresh thyme
- 3 cups of chicken broth
- ½ cup of coconut milk
- ½ tsp of sea salt
- 1 tsp of pepper

Directions:

1. Take out a large saucepan and place it onto a burner set for high heat.

2. Add your tablespoon of coconut oil, followed by your cup of chopped onions, your tsp of chopped garlic, your ½ cup of chopped mushrooms, your tsp of fresh thyme, and your 3 cups of chicken broth.

3. Stir and cook all of your ingredients together for about 15 minutes, before reducing heat to medium and adding in your ½ cup of coconut milk, your ½ tsp of sea salt, and your tsp of pepper.

4. Now stir and cook for about 5 more minutes before serving.

Pecan, Crab, and Apple Salad

When people think of salads, they probably consider Caesar and Chicken as the main draws, but this Pecan, Crab, and Apple Salad provides such a tremendous kick of flavor, you will be instantly convinced!

Prep Time: 5 min

Passive Time: 0 min

Cook Time: 0 min

Total: 5 min

Serves: 1-2

Ingredients:
- 1 cup of crabmeat
- 2 cups of diced, unpeeled apples
- ¼ cup of pecans
- ¼ cup of chopped scallions
- 1 tablespoon of chopped dill
- 2 tablespoons of lemon juice
- ½ tsp of salt
- 1 tsp of pepper

Directions:

1. Deposit your cup of crabmeat, your 2 cups of diced unpeeled apples, your ¼ cup of pecans, your ¼ cup of chopped scallions, your tablespoon of chopped dill, your 2 tablespoons of lemon juice, your ½ tsp of salt, your tsp of pepper.

2. Lightly toss these ingredients together, and serve when ready.

Rich Fish Soup

You'll feel like a million bucks when you eat this soup!

Prep Time: 5 min

Passive Time: 0 min

Cook Time: 15 min

Total: 20 min

Serves: 1-2

Ingredients:

- 2 tsp of olive oil
- ½ cup of chopped onion
- ½ tsp of chopped garlic
- 1 cup of diced tomato
- ¼ cup of diced carrots
- ¼ cup of diced celery
- ½ cup of white wine
- 1 cup of water
- ¼ tsp of grated lemon zest
- ½ pound of fresh cod
- ¼ tsp of sea salt
- 1 tsp of pepper
- 1 tablespoon of chopped parsley

Directions:

1. Add your 2 tsp of olive oil to a medium sized saucepan, and set the burner to high heat.

2. Now add your ½ cup of chopped onion, your ½ tsp of chopped garlic, your cup of diced tomato, your ¼ cup of diced carrots, and your ¼ cup of diced celery.

3. Stir and cook these ingredients for about 5 minutes before adding your ½ cup of white wine and your cup of water to the mix.

4. Now add your ¼ tsp of grated lemon zest, followed by your ½ pound of fresh cod.

5. Vigorously stir everything together for about 10 minutes.

6. Finally, season the mixture with your ¼ tsp of sea salt, your tsp of pepper, and your tablespoon of chopped parsley.

7. Serve whenever you are ready to do so.

Apples, Cherries, and Kale Salad

Kale salad with just the right blend of apples and cherries—seasoned to perfection!

Prep Time: 5 min

Passive Time: 0 min

Cook Time: 0 min

Total: 5 min

Serves: 1-2

Ingredients:
- 1 bunch of kale
- ½ cup of chopped parsley
- 1 cup of diced apples
- ½ cup of fresh pitted cherries
- ¼ cup of shaved red onion
- ½ tsp of salt
- 2 tsp of pepper

Directions:
1. Chop up your kale and place them inside a salad bowl.
2. Now add your ½ cup of chopped parsley, your cup of diced apples, your ½ cup of fresh

pitted cherries, your ¼ cup of shaved red onion, your ½ tsp of salt, and your 2 tsp of pepper to the bowl.

3. Toss ingredients together and serve.

Quick and Easy Squash Soup

As the title just might imply, this meal is quick and easy to make—but it's also delicious!

Prep Time: 0 min

Passive Time: 0 min

Cook Time: 0 min

Total: 0 min

Serves: 1-2

Ingredients:
- 1 tablespoon of olive oil
- 1 cup of chopped onions
- 1 cup of chopped squash
- 2 cups of chicken broth
- ½ tsp of nutmeg
- ¼ tsp of salt
- 1 tsp of pepper

Directions:
1. Deposit your tablespoon of olive oil into a large saucepan, before adding your cup of chopped onions, your cup of chopped squash, your 2 cups of chicken broth, your ½ tsp of

nutmeg, your ¼ tsp of salt, and your tsp of pepper.
2. Stir everything together well and cook for 15 minutes under high heat.
3. Serve when ready!

Chinese Chicken Salad

Grilled Chicken and Chinese Cabbage come together like no other!

Prep Time: 5 min

Passive Time: 0 min

Cook Time: 0 min

Total: 5 min

Serves: 1-2

Ingredients:
- 1 cup of chopped chicken breast
- 4 cups of shredded Chinese cabbage
- 1 cup of snow peas
- 1 cup of mung bean sprouts
- ½ cup of shredded carrots
- ½ cup of chopped scallions
- 1 tablespoon of chopped almonds

Directions:
1. Use a fork to shred your chopped chicken, and deposit them into a medium sized bowl, followed by your 4 cups of shredded Chinese cabbage, your cup of snow peas, your cup of mung bean sprouts, your ½ cup of shredded

carrots, your ½ cup of chopped scallions, and your tablespoon of chopped almonds.

2. Toss the salad well and serve with whatever kind of dressing you like.

Side of Veggie Chili

Have a hearty Side of Veggie Chili to go with all of that weight loss!

Prep Time: 4 min

Passive Time: 0 min

Cook Time: 25 min

Total: 29 min

Serves: 1-2

Ingredients:
1. 1 cup of black soybeans
2. 2 tablespoons of coconut oil
3. 3 tablespoons of butter
4. ½ cup of chopped onion
5. 2 tablespoons of chili powder
6. 1 tsp of dried oregano
7. 1 cup of diced tomatoes
8. ½ cup of chicken broth

Directions:
1. Place your frying pan onto a burner set for medium heat.

2. Add your 2 tablespoons of coconut oil, followed by your 3 tablespoons of butter to the pan.

3. Next, add your 2 tablespoons of chili powder and your tsp of dried oregano.

4. Stir for 2 minutes before adding in your cup of black soybeans, followed by your ½ cup of chopped onion, your cup of diced tomatoes, and your ½ cup of chicken broth.

5. Stir and cook for about 25 minutes.

6. Serve when ready.

Cauliflower Mashed Potatoes

Mashed Potatoes have always been a favorite of mine, but with all of those pesky carbs, it just isn't fasting material. But all you have to do is substitute those carb heavy potatoes for relatively carb free cauliflower and you can dig in right!

Prep Time: 4 min

Passive Time: 0 min

Cook Time: 18 min

Total: 22 min

Serves: 2-3

Ingredients:
- 1 cup of chopped cauliflower
- 2 tablespoons of heavy cream
- 2 tablespoons of melted butter
- 1 tablespoon of mayonnaise
- ½ tsp of salt

Directions:
1. Set your oven to 375 degrees.
2. While your oven is heating up, place your cup of chopped cauliflower into a heat resistant bowl followed by your 2 tablespoons of water, drizzled over the surface of the cauliflower

just to make sure that they maintain moisture.

3. Cook in the microwave for about 3 minutes.

4. Now take out of the microwave, and deposit cauliflower into a blender, followed by your 2 tablespoons of heavy cream, your tablespoon of mayonnaise, and your ½ tsp of salt.

5. Blend for about 1 minute before pouring the blended ingredients into your casserole dish.

6. Drizzle your 2 tablespoons of melted butter on top and stick the dish into the oven.

7. Cook for 15 minutes.

8. Serve when ready.

Thick and Chunky Salsa

Get out your chips, because this salsa is ready to dip!

Prep Time: 0 min

Passive Time: 0 min

Cook Time: 0 min

Total: 0 min

Serves: 2-3

Ingredients:
- ½ cup of chopped onion
- 1 tablespoon of chopped garlic
- ¼ cup of chopped jalapeno
- ½ cup of chopped tomatoes
- 1 tsp of cilantro
- 1 tablespoon of lime juice
- ¼ tsp of kosher salt

Directions:
1. Get out a blender and add your ½ cup of chopped onion, your tablespoon of chopped garlic, your ¼ cup of chopped jalapeno, your ½ cup of chopped tomatoes, your tsp of cilantro, your tablespoon of lime juice, and your ¼ tsp of kosher salt.

2. Now pulse ingredients in the blender 4 or 5 times, so that its blended but still nice and thick.

3. After this has been accomplished pour your salsa into a bowl and serve.

Chile Con Queso

This tasty recipe takes Tex Mex to the next level!

Prep Time: 5 min

Passive Time: 0 min

Cook Time: 5 min

Total: 10 min

Serves: 4-5

Ingredients:
- 1 cup of white cheddar cheese
- ½ cup of mozzarella cheese
- 2 tablespoons of heavy cream
- ½ cup of chicken broth
- ¼ cup of diced tomatoes
- 3 tablespoons of diced green chili
- ½ tsp of cumin
- 1 tsp of cayenne pepper
- 1 tablespoon of chopped cilantro

Directions:
1. Take out a medium sized saucepan and place it onto a burner set to medium heat.
2. Now add your cup of white cheddar cheese, your ½ cup of mozzarella cheese, your 2 tablespoons of heavy cream, your ½ cup of

chicken broth, your ¼ cup of diced tomatoes, your 3 tablespoons of diced green chili, your ½ tsp of cumin, your tsp of cayenne pepper, and your tablespoon of chopped cilantro.

3. Stir and cook the ingredients for about 5 minutes, thoroughly mixing the ingredients together.

4. Turn off the burner, scoop up the ingredients into a serving bowl, and your Chili Con Queso is ready for some serious dipping!

Chapter 7: Special Desserts and Beverages for Your Fast

Even during the 30-day intermittent fast challenge, there will be times in which you will crave something a little extra special. There will be times when you will want to treat yourself to a dessert or a tasty beverage. Here in this chapter we provide several recipes for healthy and tasty desserts and beverages for your fast.

Hazelnut Cookies

Crisp cookies with a hint of Hazelnut!

Prep Time: 5 min

Passive Time: 1 min

Cook Time: 15 min

Total: 21 min

Serves: 3-4

Ingredients:
- 1 cup of oat flour
- ½ cup of chopped hazelnuts
- ½ cup of white rice flour
- ½ tsp of baking powder
- 2 sticks of unsalted butter
- 2 tablespoons of sugar
- 3 tablespoons of raspberry jam
- 1 egg

Directions:
1. Set your oven's temperature for 350 degrees, and place parchment onto a cooking sheet.
2. While your oven warms up, get out a medium sized mixing bowl and add your cup of oat

flour, your ½ cup of chopped hazelnuts, your ½ cup of white rice flour, and your ½ tsp of baking powder, stirring the ingredients together well.

3. Now get out a separate bowl and add your 2 sticks of unsalted butter, and your 2 tablespoons of sugar, stir these ingredients together with an electric mixer.

4. Next add your egg, and beat with your electric mixer.

5. Now take your mixing bowl of the oat flour mixture and pour it into your bowl of egg mixture.

6. Stir these ingredients with your electric mixer until they constitute one uniform batter.

7. Now take an ice cream scoop and use it to dig out clumps of the batter and place them on your cooking sheet.

8. Place the cooking sheet in the oven and cook for about 15 minutes.

9. Once cooked allow to cool off for about 1 minute before serving.

Chocolate Chip Cookies

You'll enjoy every single chip!

Prep Time: 5 min

Passive Time: 30 seconds

Cook Time: 55 min

Total: 1 hour and 30 seconds

Serves: 3-4

Ingredients:
- 4 eggs
- 3 tablespoons of brown sugar
- 1 tablespoon of regular sugar
- 8 tablespoons of butter
- 2 tsp of vanilla extract
- 3 tablespoons of all-purpose wheat flour
- ½ cup of gluten flour
- 2 tablespoons of crude wheat bran
- 1 tsp of baking powder
- ½ cup of whole almond meal trace salt
- ½ cup of chocolate chips
- ¼ cup of chopped walnuts

Directions:

1. Go ahead and set your oven to 350 degrees.

2. While your oven is warming up, take out a medium sized mixing bowl and add your 4 eggs, your 3 tablespoons of brown sugar, and your tablespoon of regular sugar, take an egg beater and stir them together well.

3. Now add your 8 tablespoons of butter, your 2 tsp of vanilla extract, your 3 tablespoons of all-purpose wheat flour, your ½ cup of gluten flour, your 2 tablespoons of crude wheat bran, your tsp of baking powder, your ½ cup of whole almond meal trace salt, and begin beating the mixture together once again.

4. Finally, stir the chocolate chips and walnuts into the mix, place into a refrigerator, and allow to chill for about 45 minutes.

5. After 45 minutes have passed, take out of the fridge, and use your (clean) hands to shape the cookie dough into small balls.

6. Evenly space these dough balls out onto a greased cooking sheet.

7. Bake in the oven for about 10 minutes.

8. Allow to cool for about 30 seconds and serve!

Cream Cheese Cake

Get ready to bake, because this cream cheese is perfectly placed in this Cream Cheese Cake!

Prep Time: 5 min

Passive Time: 0 min

Cook Time: 30 min

Total: 35 min

Serves: 6-8

Ingredients:
- 20 ounces of cream cheese
- 4 eggs
- 2 tsp of lemon juice
- 2 tsp of vanilla extract
- 1 tablespoon of whole wheat flour
- ½ cup of sour cream

Directions:
1. Set your oven to 325 degrees.
2. As your oven heats up, get out a medium sized mixing bowl and add your 20 ounces of cream cheese, and your 4 eggs, and use an egg beater to beat the ingredients together into one uniform batter.

3. Pour this batter into a springform baking pan, and place it into your oven.

4. Cook for about 30 minutes.

5. Serve when ready.

Coconut Macaroon Cookies

Another great batch of cookies that taste great but won't upset your fast!

Prep Time: 5 min

Passive Time: 30 seconds

Cook Time: 10 min

Total: 15 min and 30 seconds

Serves: 4-5

Ingredients:
- 4 eggs
- 2 tablespoons of brown sugar
- 4 tablespoons of butter
- 2 tsp of vanilla extract
- 2 tsp of grated lemon peel
- 1 tablespoon of wheat gluten flour
- 1 tablespoon of whole wheat flour
- 1 tsp of baking powder
- 2 cups of dried coconut
- ½ cup of whole almond meal

Directions:

1. Set your oven temperature to 350 degrees.

2. As your oven heats up, get out a medium sized mixing bowl and deposit your 4 eggs, 2 tablespoons of brown sugar, and 4 tablespoons of butter.

3. Use an electric mixer to beat these ingredients together into one uniform batter.

4. Next, add your 2 tsp of vanilla extract, your 2 tsp of grated lemon peel, your tablespoon of wheat gluten flour, your tablespoon of whole wheat flour, and your tsp of baking powder, beating these ingredients into the batter as well.

5. Now take your (clean) hands and use them to fold in the 2 cups of dried coconut and your ½ cup of whole almond meal.

6. Once you have done this, take a small ice cream scooper, and use it to scoop out balls of dough.

7. Space these balls of dough out onto the surface of a greased cooking sheet and place them into the oven

8. Cook for about 10 minutes, take out, allow 30 seconds to cool, and serve.

Lean Green Smoothie

If at any point during your 30 Day Intermittent Fast Challenge you need a pick me up, look no further than this Lean Green Smoothie!

Prep Time: 3 min

Passive Time: 0 min

Cook Time: 2 min

Total: 5 min

Serves: 5-6

Ingredients:
- 1 cup of coconut milk
- 2 cups of chopped kale
- 1 cup of diced cucumber
- ½ cup of chopped avocado
- 1 tablespoon of lemon juice
- 1 tablespoon of orange juice

Directions:
1. Add your cup of coconut milk, your 2 cups of chopped kale, your cup of chopped cucumber, your ½ cup of chopped avocado, your tablespoon of lemon juice, and your tablespoon of orange juice to a blender and hit the blend button.

2. Blend for about 2 minutes before pouring yourself a glass.

Chocolate Peanut Butter Shake

You can compare this tasty recipe with the very similar beverage currently being sold at the fast food restaurant Steak and Shake. The ingredients used here are much healthier than the Steak and Shake variety however, so you can indulge in this one without wrecking your fast!

Prep Time: 2 min and 45 seconds

Passive Time: 0 min

Cook Time: 0 min

Total: 2 min and 45 seconds

Serves: 2-3

Ingredients:
- 2 cups of water
- ½ cup of coconut milk
- 2 tablespoons of "Whey Protein"
- 2 tablespoons of MCT oil
- 2 tablespoons of peanut butter
- 2 tablespoons of cacao powder

Directions:

1. Add your 2 cups of water, ½ cup of coconut milk, your 2 tablespoons of "Whey Protein", your 2 tablespoons of MCT oil, your 2 tablespoons of peanut butter, and your 2 tablespoons of cacao powder to a blender and hit the blend button.

2. Blend the ingredients for about 45 seconds.

3. Just pour blended mixture into some cups and its ready to serve.

Conclusion: Intermittent Fasting Can Change Your Life

If you are trying to lose weight and looking for a way to change your lifestyle, finding the right path to follow in the bewildering wilderness of diet plans can be frustrating. But as I hope you have learned during the course of reading this book—Intermittent fasting is not a diet fad. Intermittent fasting is *diet fact!* Because it has been scientifically proven that an intermittent dieting regimen can completely reset the body's metabolic process, and encourage the burning of fat depossits.

By holding fast (no pun intended) to the fasting regimen, recipes, and meal plans presented in this guide, you will soon see your whole lifestyle begin to change. You will not only lose that stubborn belly fat, you will also completely reinvent and reinvigorate yourself in the process. It will change your life! Thank you for reading! And good luck on your 30 Day Intermittent Fasting Challenge!

CPSIA information can be obtained
at www.ICGtesting.com
Printed in the USA
LVHW111045071019
633401LV00006B/1366/P